Natural Healing through Grains and Cereals

Healing yourself with Beans and Lentils

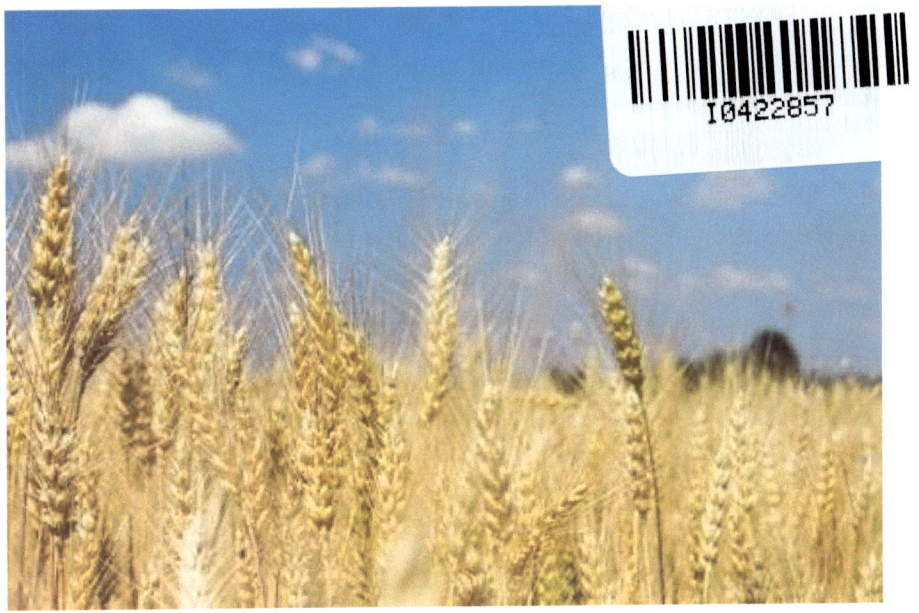

Dueep Jyot Singh

Healthy Living Series

Mendon Cottage Books

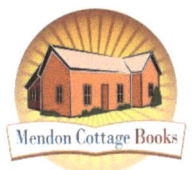

JD-Biz Publishing

Our books are available at

1 Amazon.com

2. Barnes and Noble

3. Itunes

4. Kobo

5. Smashwords

6. Google Play Books

Table of Contents

Introduction

Since ancient times, man has known the value of cereals like wheat, maize, rice, barley, oats, and millet in order to make his daily bread. Apart from the nutritive value of all the cereals, and grains, they are necessary to keep the body healthy and functioning properly.

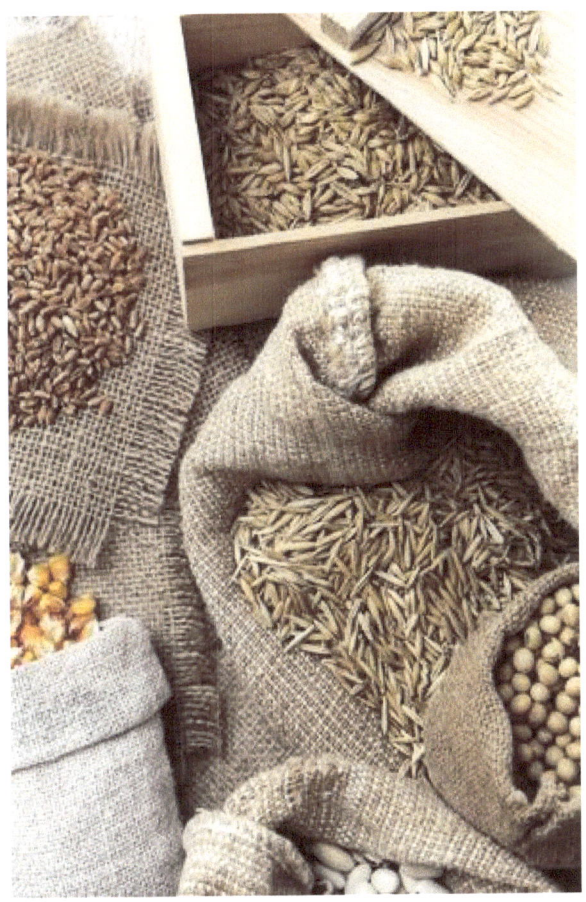

This book is going to tell you all about the curative properties of most of the grains we eat. Naturally, wheat is one of the most well-known of the grains which mankind knows for centuries, and bread and meat has been the staple diet of many societies, for millenniums, with a little bit of greens on the side.

Wheatgrass has long been known as one of the most powerful natural health giving ingredients known to man. In the same way, sprouted grains, as well as sprouted beans, like mung sprouts have for a long time giving man an extra supportive source of natural protein, minerals, vitamins, and other natural healing and restorative elements.

Barley – Hordeum vulgare

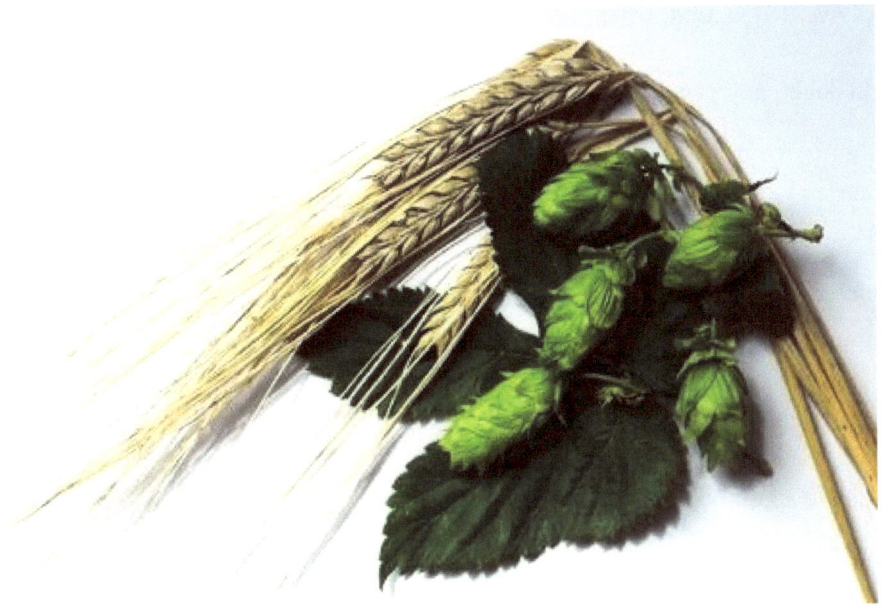

Barley with hops – the main ingredients for making beer

Barley is a high-fiber Hardy grain/cereal, which is normally used for stock feed, and for brewing purposes. Once upon a time in medieval times, the people in many parts of Europe existed on barley. Even today, barley is the staple diet in Tibet. The staple food of this area is called Tsampa which is made out of roasted barley. Even though we were not near Tibet when we were holidaying in Ladakh, way back in the late 80s, we asked our host if we could manage to get some Tsampa to eat.

It has a nutty sort of flavor. The making of the Tsampa is a laborious process. You are going to dry the barley, after washing it extensively. After that, you roasted the seeds. Traditionally, it is roasted in a very hot sand, and after I had has been roasted, it is sieved so that all the sand grains are removed through the sieve. This roasted grain is then ground, and whenever you want to eat it, you can mix it with buttered tea to have a ready convenience food, whenever you want it.

In Tibet, any person suffering from a burn would have that area treated with a paste of tsampa and ground cumin seeds. In other parts of the world, the barley would be roasted and then ground to obtain barley oil. This oil was then used to treat the burned area. But taking out oil is a very cumbersome process, so I would rather suggest using ground barley with cumin seeds. Easy to grind, easy to apply for natural curative results.

Barley for Beauty

I have a number of Tibetan friends who have this perfectly glowing skin. Apart from eating lots of tsampa which gives them plenty of protein and natural nutrients, they use this barley as a face scrub.

So if you want a clear complexion, glowing skin, or to just get rid of that oily skin, just take some barley flour, 2 tablespoons full and add 2 tablespoons full of milk to it. You can add a little bit of honey, a little bit of turmeric, or a little bit of mustard oil to it. All of these are antiseptic and curative. Now apply this all over your body as a scrub, instead of soap.

I tried it a couple of days ago, especially now that the winter is coming in. When I came out of my hot shower, I was thrilled at the silky feel of the skin, and I did not even need to apply any moisturizing lotion afterwards, because the milk and the honey had done all the moisturizing. You have to have a hot bath or shower with this scrub, because that is what has the most positive effect on your skin.

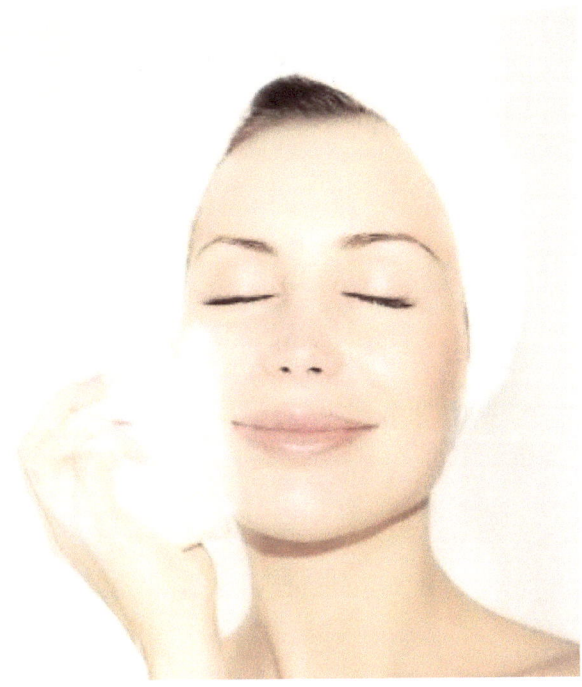

Here is another little-known use to which barley has been put by our ancestors. This is a skin whitener. So if you have a dusky complexion or you want to lighten your skin even more, take two teaspoonfuls of fresh milk cream, and add a tablespoon of barley flour to it. Make a paste of it with a little bit of water and use it as a scrub, all over your face and hands to whiten the texture of the skin, and give it a lighter tone. Just like oatmeal, it is also a well known skin whitening product, but somehow this particular use got lost in the flood of knowledge, in the 21st-century. Here it is again.

Diabetes

This cure was given to me by a naturopath, who incidentally suffers from diabetes. So he keeps on looking for natural remedies from all over the world, including bitter gourd juice. According to him, this was a remedy told to him by an Egyptian friend which worked for him.

You may want to try it out. Take 5 pounds of barley, half a pound of Bengal Gram – Cicer arietinum, 1 pound of soybean, 1 pound of fenugreek seeds, and 1 pound of wheat. – That means you have 8 ½ pounds of the most nourishing and healing grains in the world today. Grind them all together, and use them for bread. This is one of the best ways in order to cure and control your diabetes. Naturally, in many parts of Asia, the bread is made into "tortillas"– also known as roti. Even stuffed breads can be made from this particular flour.

Even if you are not suffering from diabetes, any food item with Bengal gram is going to be healthy and nourishing. You may want to try it out just to keep healthy.

Asthma

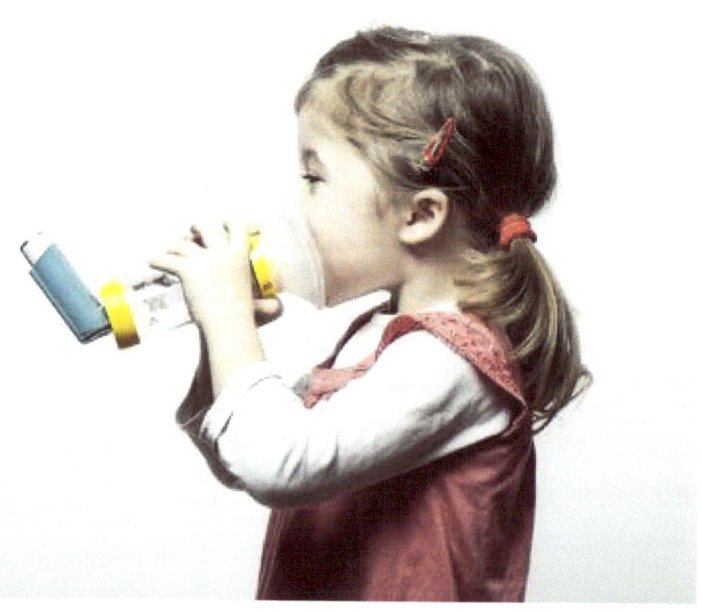

This is a natural remedy for all those people suffering from asthma, and taking drugs with terrible side effects. If you are one of those people, my sympathies are with you, and it is time you threw away your inhaler, and lived life on a precipice.

This is a natural remedy, which is a time-tested cure for asthma. Firstly, you are going to make some barley ash. This is done by putting it in an earthenware pot and allowing to burn. Traditionally, this is normally done by putting it in a pot, and adding red-hot coals to the mixture. This will burn the barley seeds to a crisp.

After they are burnt, cover the pot, making it airtight, and leave it for four hours. Remove the coal and grind the rest of the burnt barley. You can also roast and burn the barley by putting it on your griddle and forgetting about it!

After all, you just need burnt ash, don't you.

Once you have got this ash, you are going to take 6 g of it. That makes 1.2 teaspoons. Now add 6 g of rock candy to this ground ash. Mix these two together, and grind them up well. Drink these 12 g morning and evening with water. This is a permanent cure for asthma.

Mung Bean– Phaseolus aureus

I remember when I was a child, the moment I felt feverish, my grandmother used to restore me with a kedgeree made up of boiled rice and mung beans. Not only was this easily digestible, especially when it was eaten down with yogurt, but it was an excellent restorative also.

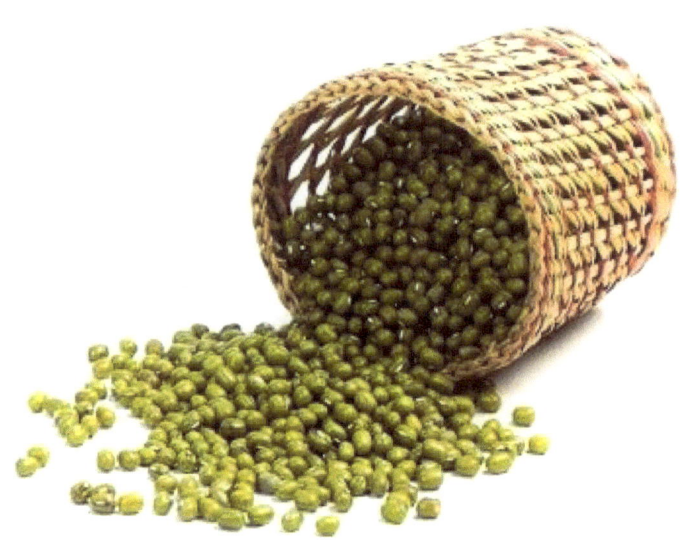

So when any person around you is suffering from fever, all you have to do is give him mung bean or any other bean soup. Do not remove the outer shell, even though these beans are also found without their outer green husk/shell.

Mung for Fever

In ancient times, this fever breaking remedy was made by cooking mung beans with dried gooseberry. Gooseberry is supposed to be the most excellent immunity system strengthening fruit ever known to man. Also, this gave the cooked mung dish a sour taste and flavor. This was fed to the patient morning and evening in order to clear his system of any infection and toxins.

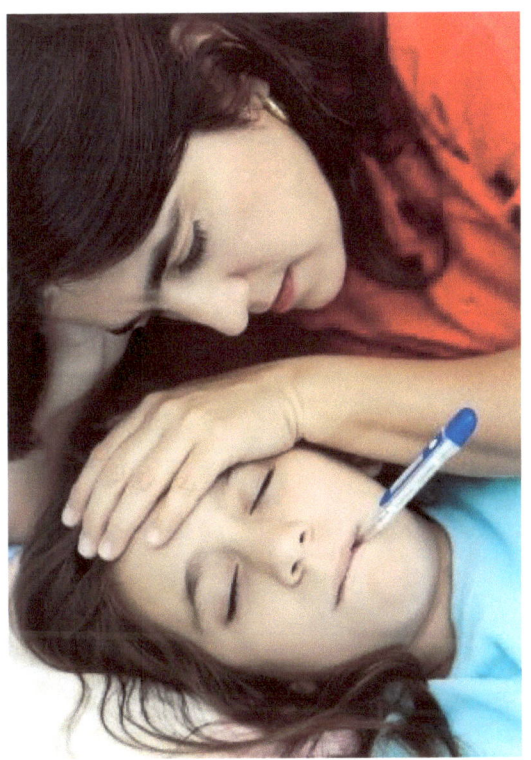

Mung for Recuperation

After a person recovered from his fever, there was going to be a couple of months before he could gain enough of energy to get back to his state of natural good health. This was when mung was given every day to the patient to restore him. For all those patients to whom the Doctor had prescribed a no cereal diet, instead, he would be given boiled mung water. This water would be filtered and salt, pepper, and mild spices of choice being added to it.

This water was given often to the patient, as a soup. It is an excellent healer, and easily digestible. It is also tasty, thanks to the salt, pepper and spices. The rest of the family could eat the boiled mung fried with onions, tomatoes, spices, and other appetite enhancing herbs.

Excessive Perspiration –Hyperhidrosis

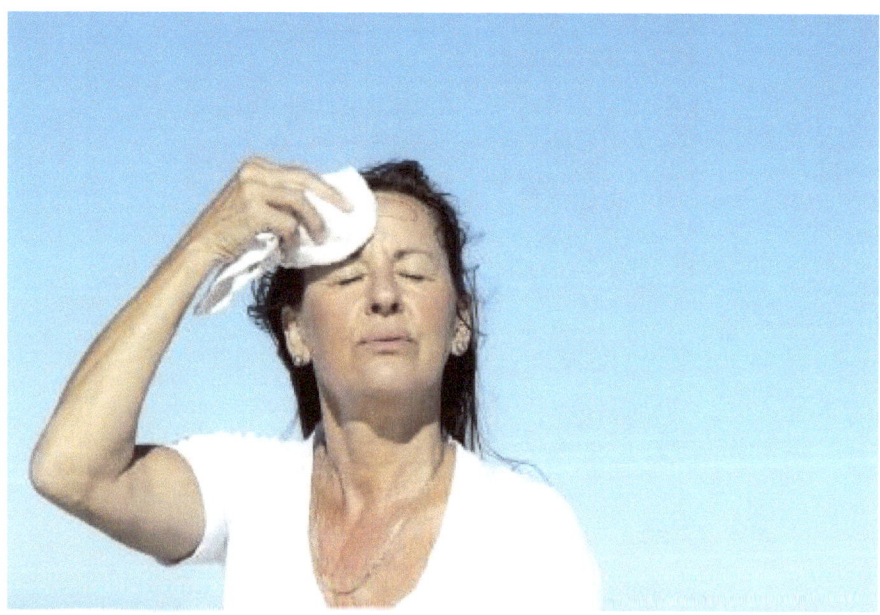

There are many people out there who suffer from a rather annoying condition known as excessive perspiration or hyperhidrosis. I did not know that I suffered from it, especially last summer, when I went out in the June heat, and soon found myself drenched as if I had been standing under a waterfall. Even excessive mopping up with a handkerchief brought no visible results because it was as if the sweat glands had started overacting.

Naturally, getting back to air-conditioned atmospheres was very detrimental to my chest, causing possible pulmonary infections. So I asked around for a natural cure for hyperhidrosis.

This is really easy. Just dry fry/roast some mung beans on a griddle pan. Then grind them into a fine powder. Use this on your face and body as a scrub. This is going to prevent and cure hyperhidrosis. It did me, along with drinking large quantities of fresh lime juice lemonade with sugar. This prevented dehydration as well as got rid of all the summer toxins.

Eczema

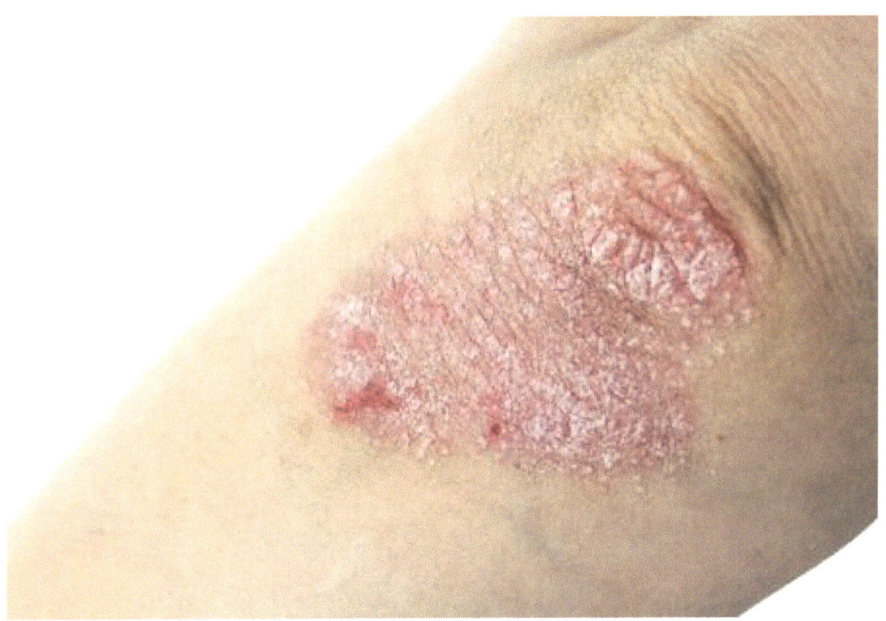

Take a fistful of mung beans and soak them in just that much amount of water, which allows itself to be absorbed in the beans. Allow to soak for two hours. Then grind the beans into a paste with a little bit more of water, and apply the paste all over the affected areas. This is good to cure Eczema and other skin problems including drying out pimples.

Constipation

In many parts of the East, even today, anybody suffering from chronic constipation is fed a breakfast of a mixture of rice and mung beans. Traditionally this is made with a proportion of 2:1 – two parts mung and one part rice. Add salt and herbs to taste. The British took this dish back to their country, as a breakfast dish, adding smoked haddock, boiled eggs, and everything else they had at hand to make this an appetizing meal for breakfast.

Kedgeree- Kichuri

This is a traditional Eastern dish, adapted for Western palates, and spread all over the world by the Britishers in their colonies the $18^{th-19th}$ century.

Traditional Khichri
[Literally mung dal hotch potch. In Britain, this dish is eaten for breakfast, with fish added, and is called kedgeree.]

One Cup - Yellow or green Moong Dal
Half Cup Basmati Rice
To Taste - Salt
5-6 Cups - Water
For Tadka/seasoning
2 Tsp - Ghee/Oil

3-4 - Green Chili

A Pinch - Asafoetida/Hing

1 tsp - Cumin Seeds/Jeera

2 tsp - Minced Garlic

Clean the rice as well as the mung and then soak it for 15 minutes. Add three cups water to the rice and the dal and allow to cook till the water is absorbed.

If you have a pressure cooker, allow it to whistle thrice. That means that this is going to be cooked into porridge consistency.

It takes a while for green mung to be cooked, so we are going to remove it from the heat and mash it up along with the rice with a spoon and a little bit of oil/ghee. [Clarified butter] Then put it on the boil again with one more cup water. This quantity is going to depend on how watery or how thick you want your porridge to be.

If you are going to be using it as comfort food, you can do the tempering. If you are going to be using it as food for invalids, just add rock salt, pepper and a little bit of lemon juice sprinkled on top, and give it to your patient with a bowl of yogurt. This is easy to digest. Do not eat it with pickles, if you are suffering from dysentery/diarrhea, and want to cure it. After you have been cured, you can eat it with anything!

Tempering is what is going to give that extra touch of yumminess to this Khichdi.

Mix the garlic with the cumin seeds and scissor the chilies. Heat the oil in your frying pan, add garlic and asafetida, and fry until it is a Golden brown. Now add the chilies and fry until you hear the crackle of the cumin.

This tempering is poured straight over the khichadi and mixed. It is then served hot with yogurt, pickles, and your favorite salads. Enjoy, because this is the most easily digested of foods.

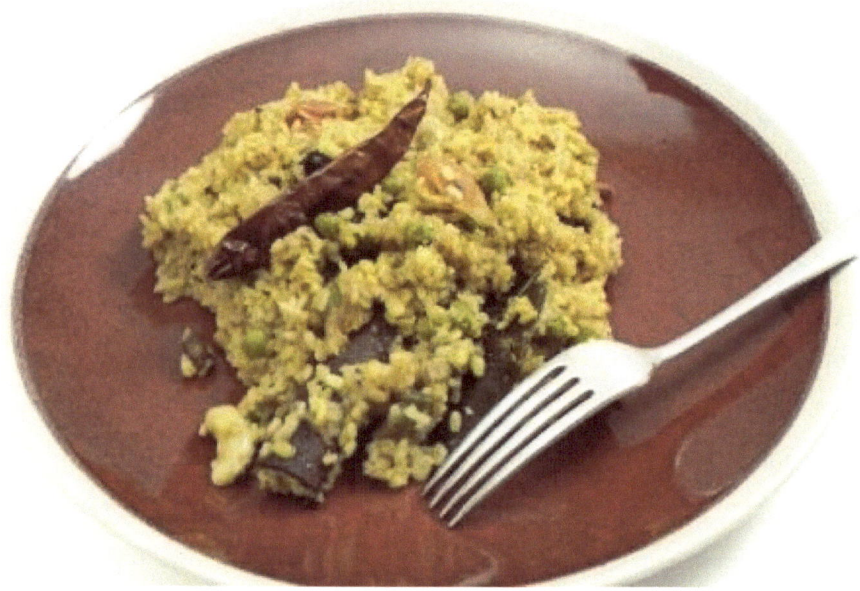

This is what the authentic tempered traditional khichuri looks like. It is hot and spicy.

Burns

Traditionally, anybody suffering from Burns would find the old wise woman of the family grinding mung with a little bit of water, mixing it with honey, and applying it all over the Burns. Not only would this take away the burning sensation but would prevent it from blistering and also cure the one without leaving any sort of scar.

How to Make Sprouts

Sprouts can be made from any beans type and variety, even though lentils like mung are the most popular traditional mediums for making this nutritious addition to your diet. To make sprouts, you are going to dip a clean piece of cloth in water and then wring it out. Take your choice of grains/pulses and spread them all over that wet and moist cloth. Cover the grains with another layer of wet and moist cloth.

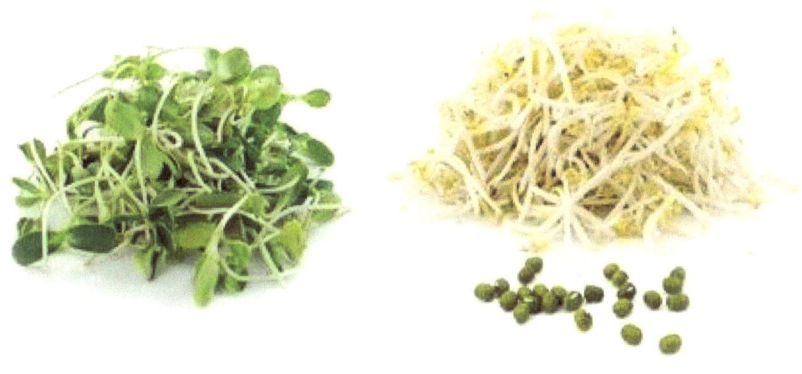

Keep for 36 – 48 hours, making sure that the water content on the cloth remains ever present because after all these seeds are germinating. After 48 hours, you are going to get sprouted grains, which can be eaten in the morning with breakfast, or whenever required.

Do not fry them in oil. If you are a heart patient, you may want to just dry stir fry in a wok and sprinkle it all over your food or add to your salad.

Wheat –Triticum vulgare

I remember at my college, starting a stunt with which all we science students managed to learn the names of the botanical plants we were studying, by calling them by their Latin names. We did that for the chemical source also. Our non-science stream friends got really tired of us asking us to pass on the sodium chloride or Triticum vulgare bread, in a display of intellectual snobbery!

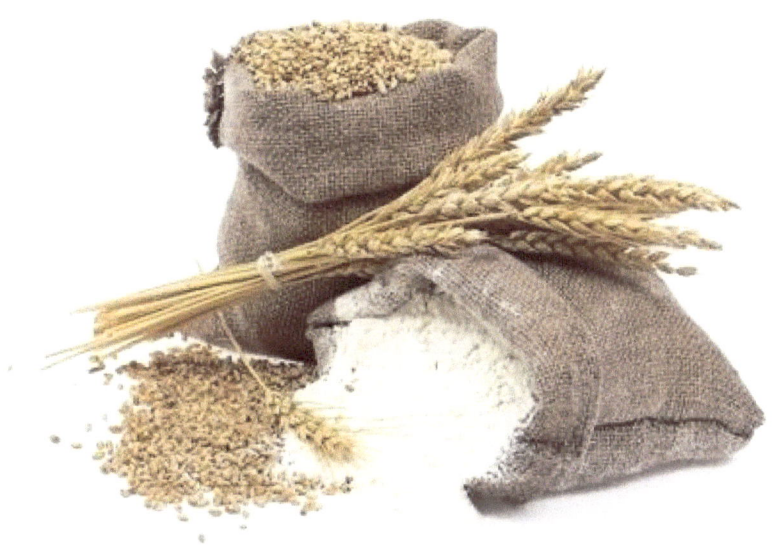

But that helped, because even more than two decades later, I have not forgotten the Latin names of the 300+ plants, I had to study belonging to 40 families.

Boils and Skin Ailments

This is a natural cure, which was done in ancient times, especially when people suffered from painful boils. They took 20 grains of wheat and chewed them to a pulp. After that, they applied that pulp to that affected area. This cured the infection.

When I told a friend, who told me this, that it was elementary my dear Watson, it was the saliva which was curing the ailment, she looked pensively at her dog licking any easily reachable part of its body and said that perhaps I had the right idea. Anyway, this is the natural poultice for painful infected boils, especially in the rainy season or when you drink polluted water.

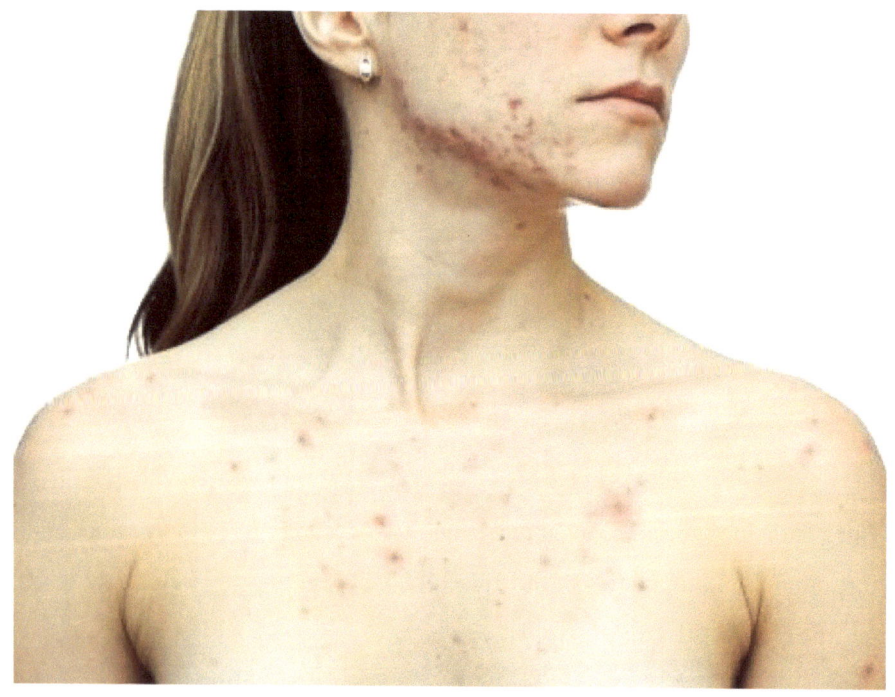

If you did not want to go through the chewing process, you could take a little bit of wheat flour, and add a little bit of salt and water to it. This was fried on a griddle pan with a little bit of water until it turned brown. This paste was then applied on the affected area, so that the infection was drawn away after the boil "ripened" with the poultice fomentation.

Apply this, three times a day, on the boil so that it comes to a head and the infection can be opened to remove the accumulated suppuration.

Diabetes Porridge

This is a porridge, which is going to cure you of diabetes. For this you need 500 g of mung, without the skin removed, 500 g of rice 500 g of wheat and 500 g of pearl millet – *Pennisetum glaucum*. Mix them all together and roast them. Now grind them to a coarse porridge.

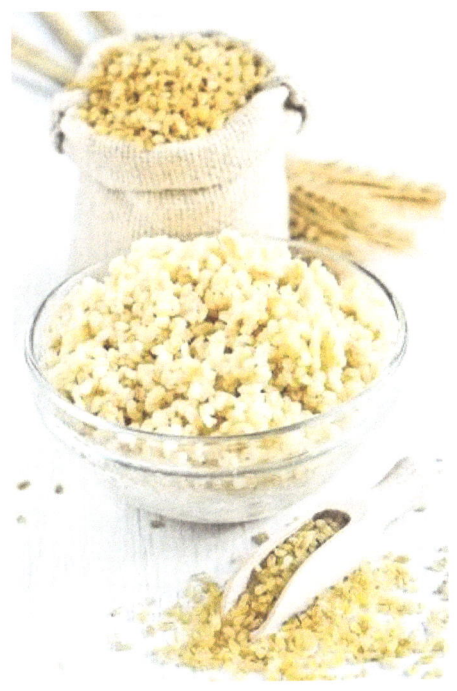

After this, you are going to add 20 g of bishops weed and 50 g of white sesame seeds to the mixture. When you have to cook it, you are going to take 50 g of this porridge, and boil it in 400 g of water. You can add rock salt, green chilies,coriander, and seasonal vegetables to this tasty porridge and eat it morning and evening for 10 days.

This is a natural cure, for those people dependent on insulin injections. It is also an excellent weight reducing porridge. It is going to get your diabetes under control.

For the rest of your life, you are going to eat this, especially if you are suffering from diabetes, you are never going to suffer from diabetes ever again.

Pain Reliever

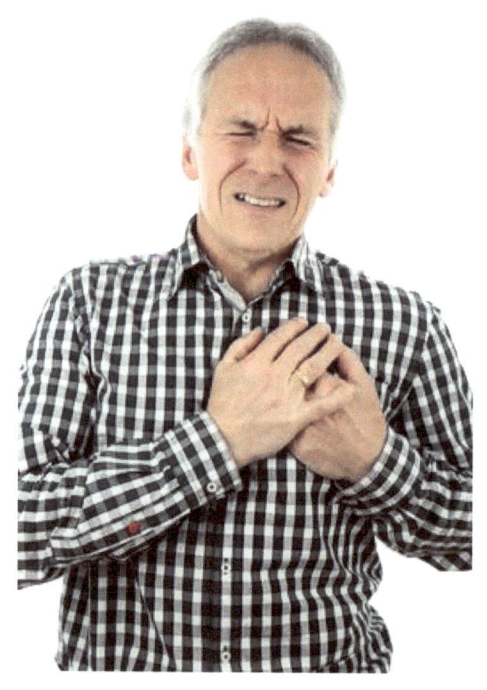

I was given this remedy by an old friend, who said that this was a pain reliever, especially from people suffering from chronic pain due to ailments. She said that it worked for her father, especially when he suffered from age-related pain.

For this, you need 3 tablespoons full of half crushed whole-wheat – normally used for making porridge also known as Bulgur in the Middle East or dalia – and soak it overnight in one cup of water. The next morning, you put two table spoonfuls of ground coriander leaves and coriander powder, two tea spoons full of poppy seeds and milk, and sugar to taste and cook this like a porridge. You can add or decrease the amounts of the ingredients, according to your requirements.

This is an excellent pain reliever and also helps in curing digestive problems. This is excellent for old people, because it gives them lots of energy.

The moment she told me this recipe, I said "Eureka, poppy seeds, meaning opium, which is a natural pain reliever," and she threw a fluffy cushion at me. She really hates my habit of being a minute dissector of why some particular ingredient is necessary to cure some particular ailment.

Call that my birthright. The Pursuit of Knowledge!

This is one used to which I put wheat flour, which may not cure you of any particular disease, but it is going to cure your home of cockroaches! Just take some equal amounts of wheat flour and boric acid. Knead them together into a dough with a little bit of water. Now make small pellets of this, and place them in any place, which you find infested with cockroaches.

The cockroaches are going to be attracted to the smell of the wheat flour and are going to get totally sterilized by the boric acid. So no cockroaches. A friend of mine laughingly told me that I should make these pellets and sell them in the market as cockroach repellents at USD.10 a packet, and she was serious. That is because our area is full of huge overgrown pestilential cockroaches.

So here is my ten cents worth of excellent cockroach repellent advice.

Urinary Problems

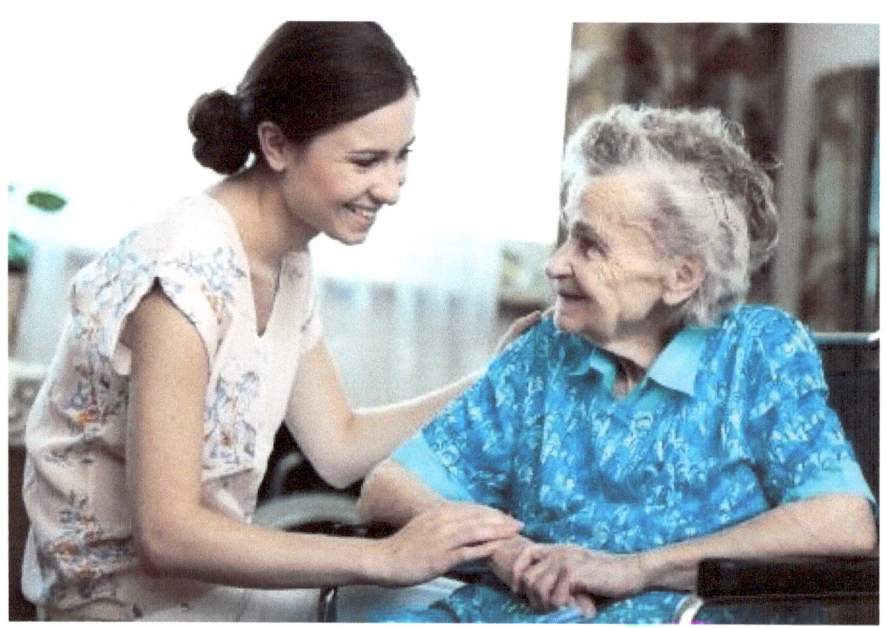

Old people suffer more often from urinary infections

If you are suffering from any sort of urinary infection, all you have to do is soak 2 teaspoons full of wheat flour or one teaspoonful of wheat seeds in 250 g of water overnight. The next morning, you are going to filter this liquid and drink it with a little bit of honey/rock candy for taste. Do this every day, once a day, until your urinary infection is cured.

Sprouted Wheat

Sprouted wheat is rich in vitamin E. This is an excellent source of energy and good health. They are excellent to strengthen your immunity system. Thanks to the large amount of vitamins present in them. According to Hippocratus, your food is what heals you wheatgrass juice is one of the most excellent natural foods, which you can drink. Along with the large amount of chlorophyll, which you are going to be ingesting, you are eating natural greens, especially when they are sprouted.

In fact, some years ago, researchers in Boston decided to try wheatgrass remedies to cure people suffering from diabetes, asthma, allergies, and skin diseases. They found a very positive percentage of these diseases being cured through a wheatgrass diet.

If you want to know more about the curative properties of wheatgrass, here is one of our publications showing you how wheatgrass can help cure you naturally.

http://www.amazon.com/Miracle-Wheatgrass-keep-you-healthy-ebook/dp/B00QH00X86/ref=sr_1_1?ie=UTF8&qid=1445476438&sr=8-1&keywords=wheatgrass+book+davidson

Wheatgrass Juice

Here is how you are going to make wheatgrass juice out of sprouted wheat. Firstly, you are going to grow it. Take 12 wooden boxes or even bamboo baskets – I am talking about containers in which you can grow wheatgrass on your terrace. Now put some fertilized soil in these boxes and label them from one to 12. Do not over fertilize the soil, in the initial stages because too much of rich organic material is too strong for these baby seeds.

Every day, you are going to put in a fistful of wheat seeds, turn by turn, in all the boxes. So by the 12th day, you are going to see lots of wheat sprouts inbox number one, ready for harvesting. This grows best in the shade. Keep watering them at regular intervals.

The sprouts are going to spring up within 3 to 4 days within 8 to 10 days, you are going to get sprouts of 7 to 8 inches in height. You are going to harvest these plants by uprooting them from the root.

Remove the root and wash the rest of the plant with its tender green leaves and stalk. This is now known as wheatgrass. Grind it in your food grinder with a little bit of water.

Prepare half a glass of this water and give this to the patient, first thing in the morning on an empty stomach.

Do the same thing – half a glass – given to the patient in the evening. Do not allow him to eat anything for two hours afterwards or before.

After this glass of juice, give him fresh soup of green vegetables. The food should be simple without spices. Boiled, steamed, roasted, baked foodstuffs, or foodstuffs prepared in any way without frying in oil are excellent food items to be given to the patient.

You are going to see a visible effect within the next 10 – 15 days. This is the reason why wheatgrass is called green blood, because it rejuvenates your blood and system and makes you feel healthy again.

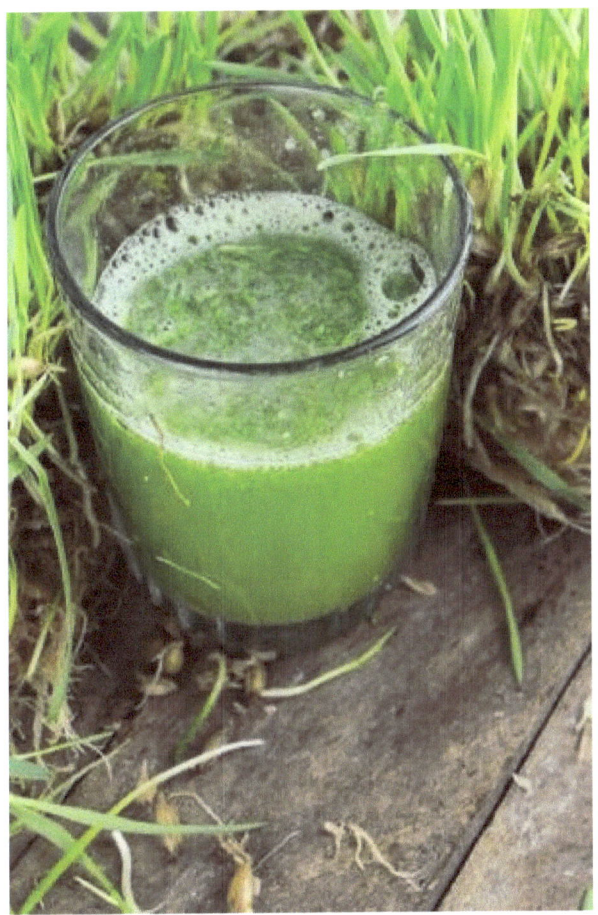

It is going to take you 2 to 3 months to cure a serious and chronic ailment. When you take out the juice, and filter it, do not throw away the green ground wheatgrass. Feed it to the patient with a little bit of salt and pepper.

 If you do not want to go through the trouble of reducing it, you can scissor the wheatgrass into small pieces, and eat it with your meals as an extra salad. This goes well with raw vegetables and green leafy vegetables. But remember not to eat any fruit along with this salad.

Make sure that the sprouts do not grow more than 8 inches in height. Remember to keep renewing these seeds in the boxes as you harvest their harvest, so that they are ready for harvesting on the 13th day.

The juices always fed to the patient fresh. That is because the potency is going to get lost, the more you keep it. If you feed it to the patient after three hours, it is going to be of absolutely no use at all.

Precautions

Drink 50 mL of this juice, slowly and sip by sip, in the beginning. After that, you can increase the quantity slowly. For chronic cases, naturopaths may give you as much of 300 mL.

Make sure that you do not adulterate any of these doses with fresh fruit juice. I saw one of my friends doing this, and I told her why she was counteracting the power of wheatgrass juice with orange juice. According to her, she was getting the benefit of both at the same time. According to me, she was counteracting the effect of both, by mixing up fruit juice with wheatgrass juice. Both are definitely not compatible.

Instead, she could add freshly ground mint leaves or any sort of green leafy vegetables like spinach to this juice. This would support the power of wheatgrass. Also, I told her not to add any extra additives in order to get some extra taste boost. This included salt, spices, and lemons. These are a no-no when you are drinking wheatgrass juice.

Along with drinking this wheatgrass juice, you can add another protein and energy support booster. This is done by taking half a cup of wheat, putting it into cups of water and leaving it overnight. You are going to drink one cup of this water morning evening every day. The rest of the wheat which you left overnight can be eaten, with salt-and-pepper and pieces of ginger to clear your system. Or you can dry it and grind it for wheat flour.

Many people find themselves suffering from stomach problems, or even nausea in the initial stages of drinking wheatgrass juice. That is because their body is not accustomed to so much greenery and protein in one go. Some may suffer from diarrhea or feel cold. Do not worry, the body is just getting rid of the infection and the toxins. You are soon going to feel healthier.

In the initial stages, you are going to drink this wheatgrass juice for 40 days in order to see a visible improvement of your condition. After that, you can continue this for as long as you wish.

Wheatgrass has vitamin C, A, B, and E. Apart from that, it has hundred three essential minerals, amino acids, fiber, lipase, and other essential nutrients, necessary to keep your body healthy.

This green blood is capable of increasing the hemoglobin count in your blood. So if you are suffering from anemia, you may want to try out adding wheatgrass to your diet right now. This also is excellent for controlling cholesterol and diabetes as well as helping cure them.

Wheat Sherbet

The moment one uses the word sherbet, one is immediately visualizing lemon squash, or orange juice or any such cooling sherbet. Try this one, made of wheat.

Take about two fistfuls of organic wheat, in a clay pot, and add a glass of water to it. Allow it to rest overnight. The next morning, you are going to filter this water and add honey to it. Here is your sherbet, which you drink down on an empty stomach, first thing in the morning. This is excellent for your immune system. It is going to provide you with lots of energy. Try it out as a refreshing healing drink right now.

Wheat Husk as a Coffee Substitute!

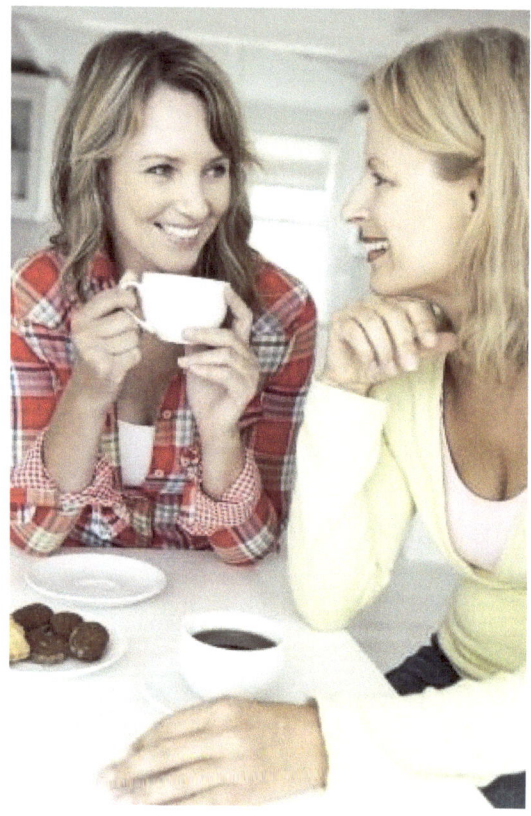

I tried this stunt on a neighbor who is a complete coffee addict. She cannot do without her daily hit of caffeine, early in the morning and often throughout the day. That year, our area was inundated with freak flash floods and nobody could move out of the neighborhood, for about five days.

And that was when her coffee supply got finished. She was in panic mode. What sort of abnormal friend was I, who did not drink tea and coffee at all, and have a little bit of coffee for her to be borrowed when in dire straits?

So I tried this stunt on her – I took some wheat husk and roasted it on the griddle, until it was red in color, but not burnt. Then I used it as a coffee substitute, with milk, sugar, and water. According to her, it was delicious and what was the brand name of that particular coffee? I think this is autosuggestion, because I took out this powder from an old bottle of coffee, which I had by chance.

She took it as "coffee" and now I am her best friend, yet once again. So for all you coffee addicts, who want to get rid of that caffeine fix, try this proteinaceous substitute. It is healthier, it is tastier, and also, it is going to cure you of blood pressure, heart attacks, constipation, flatulence, and make your body strong and healthy again.

Bengal Gram

Bengal gram or Cicer arietum is grown all over the world, and apart from it being a natural beauty enhancer, it is excellent to provide you with an immediate source of energy.

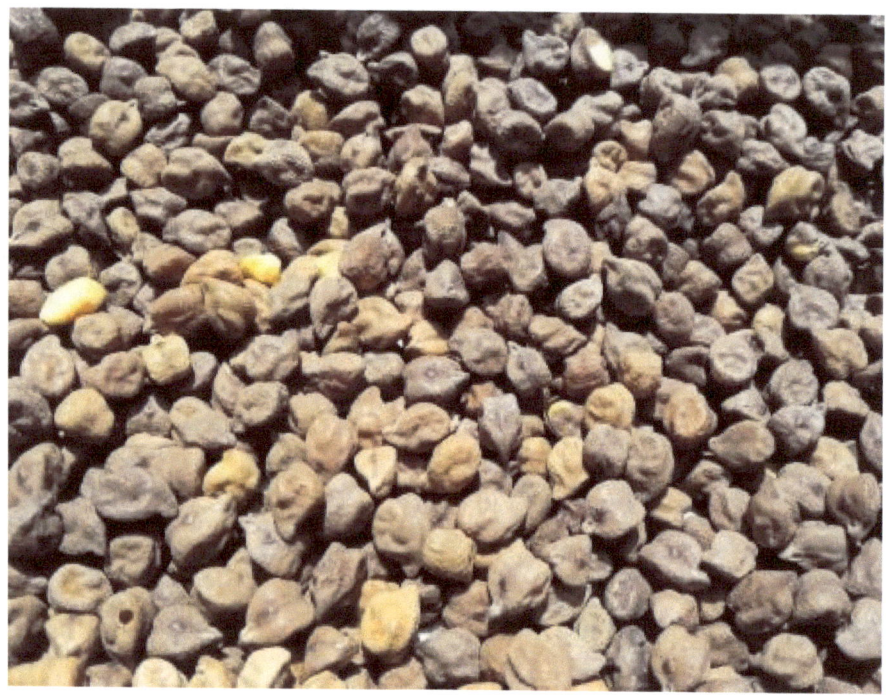

That is because Bengal gram sprouts are full of vitamin C. Have them for breakfast everyday. This is sprouted by putting the necessary amount of Bengal grams in water for 24 hours. After that, you wrap them up in a wet cloth for 20 hours. This is going to sprout them.

These Bengal gram sprouts can be eaten with lemon, minced ginger, pepper, green coriander, green chilies, rock salt, black salt, and spices, according to taste.

This breakfast is going to strengthen your lungs, increase your blood count, and clean up your blood. It also prevents and cures heart diseases and gives you plenty of energy, thanks to its natural protein.

Black gram has been given to horses for millenniums, along with oats because it is the best source of energy out there. In many parts of the world today, children are not being given expensive dry fruit to eat, but a fistful of black sprouted grams.

Constipation

Take a fistful of grams, and soak them overnight in water in the morning, grind some dried ginger and roasted cumin seeds together, and sprinkle them over the grams before eating. The water is drunk one hour after you have eaten the grams. This clears your system and gets rid of the constipation.

Dandruff

This is a time-tested cure for dandruff. Dandruff is nothing but the dried skin from your scalp and it takes seven days for one layer from your scalp to peel off, giving way to a fresh new layer of skin on your head. That is why shampoo companies tell you to use their shampoo, every seven days, and it is going to keep you dandruff free. Of course it is going to keep you dandruff free, because it takes seven days for a layer of dandruff to be formed. And shampooing it is going to remove that layer.

This is a natural way in which you are going to get rid of dandruff, instead of buying chemical-based, selenium-based shampoos. Take two large table spoons of gram flour and put it in one glass of water. Rub it all over your scalp and hair. This is a natural shampoo and you do not need to shampoo your hair with chemical shampoos ever again. This gets rid of the dandruff.

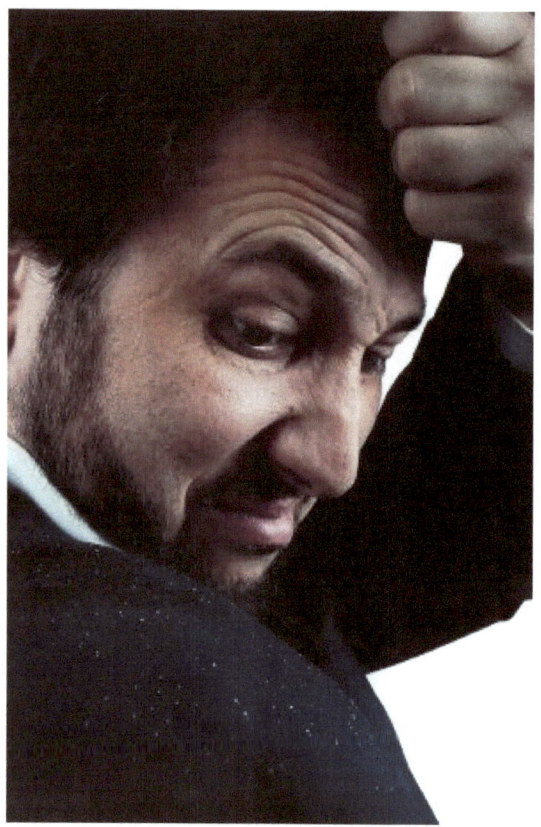

Some years ago, I saw an old lady in her 80s but still with dark hair shampooing her hair with a mixture of yogurt and gram flour. This was how her ancestors kept their hair dark and silky and soft. This shampooing was done every three days. Try this out right now.

Ascites – Abdominal Swelling

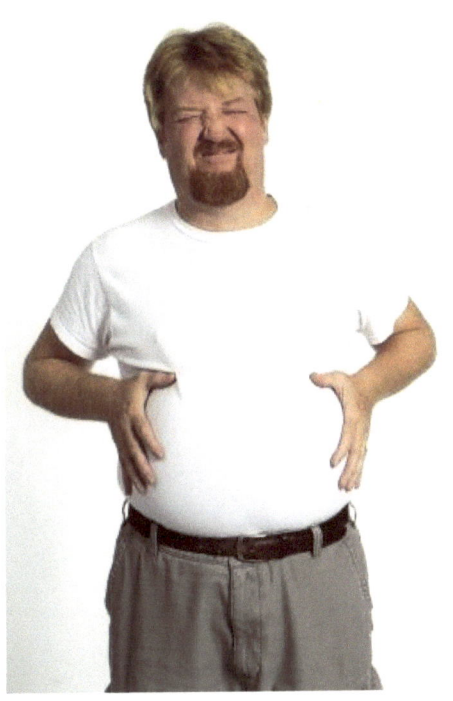

This normally happens when there is an accumulation of water in your peritoneal region. The stomach swells up. This is normally a side effect of an infection or even cancer.

If you are suffering from ascites, there is no time to be lost. Just add 25 g of Bengal gram, and heat in 250 g of water, until the water is reduced to half. Drink this water up. Do this for three weeks, to cure ascites permanently. Also, if you are suffering from a serious case of ascites, you may want to eat the Bengal gram "dal", which is shelled Bengal gram.

Bake it or cook it like you would cook beans.

Beauty Remedies

I cannot resist beauty remedies, especially when nearly every natural remedy, of which I know starts with take some Bengal gram flour. Bengal gram flour is considered to be the best dirt remover and skin exfoliator known to people in Asia. In fact, many people even today, never use soap on their bodies because of its harsh chemical content.

They just take a couple of tablespoons full of Bengal gram, mix it with a little bit of milk to make a paste and use it as a scrub to get rid of all the dirt, and leave the skin glowing.

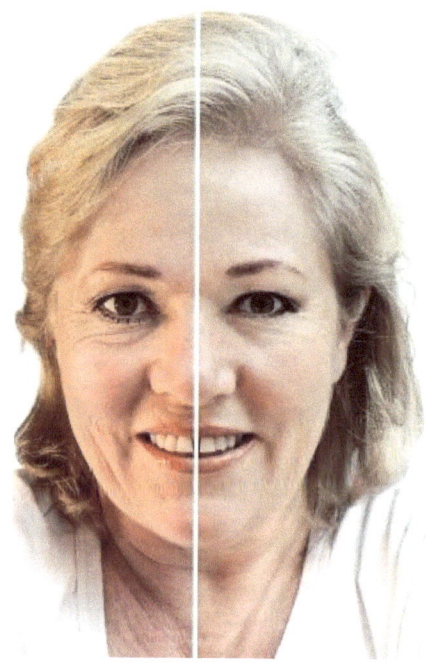

Using this as a wash on your face, and forgetting all about the chemical moisturizers, lotions and potions is going to keep your skin blemish free and soft. If you are suffering from sunburn, or suntan just take a little bit of Bengal gram flour and put it in milk or yogurt. Apply this paste all over your body morning and evening and leave it for half an hour before washing it with warm water or scrubbing it off. This is going to get rid of the suntan and sunburn.

If you have real bad skin damage, you will need to soak some Bengal gram in water overnight. After that, the next morning, you grind this and mix it with your favorite oil – olive oil, wheat germ oil, coconut oil, any moisturizing oil ready at hand, which is not chemical-based – and add a little bit of turmeric to it. The turmeric is an antiseptic and clears your skin of sunburn. Remember that turmeric is capable of staining your skin so that is why you need to remove this paste after it has dried on your skin for half an hour, with milk.

Traditionally in the East, brides were bathed by the womenfolk of the groom's family, so that they could see that the body was not deformed or had any "unlucky" marks, or moles on the body with a gram flour paste, every day for one week before the wedding.

It was not only effective enough to make the skin glow and soft, but you can use this as a full body cleanser before you have your shower every day and see all that dirt and grime slough away.

For this you need a tablespoons full of gram flour, 5 tablespoons of yogurt, 5 tablespoons full of milk, and 3 tablespoons full of turmeric powder. The bridal mixture had saffron and powdered almonds in it, but I do not intend to make up that traditional expensive mixture.

Rub this all over your body and face. Leave on for 10 minutes, and then start rubbing slowly in circular motions. This is going to get rid of the dirt and the dead cells. Then have your shower when you are completely scrubbed.

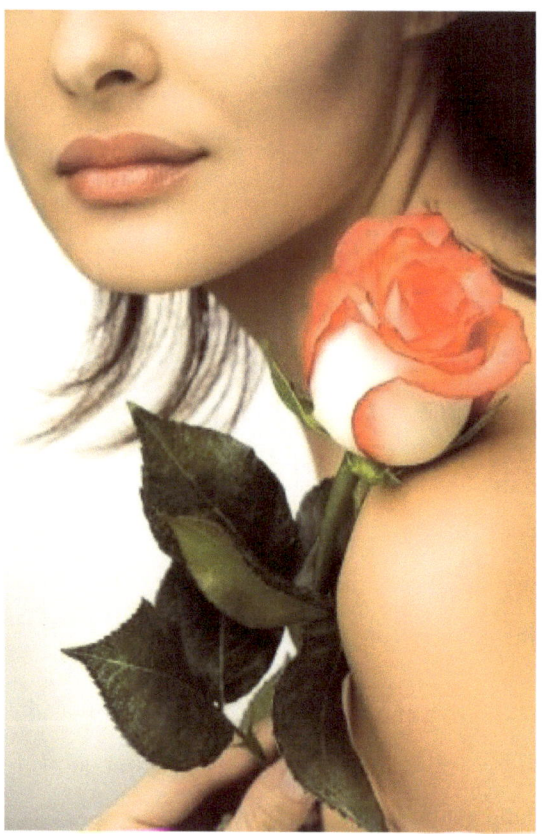

Do this every day, if you can. Apart from having a soft, silky and wrinkle free skin, you may find yourself throwing out your soaps and expensive moisturizing lotions. The moisturizing is done with the milk and with yogurt. The turmeric is an excellent antibiotic. In fact, if you want to feel younger than your age, try this out right now. You will never "look" 50, 60, or 70 again!

Incidentally, this paste is excellent to get rid of itching and other skin diseases.

Leucoderma

This is a mineral deficiency ailment where the patient is going to see white spots and patches appearing on his body. The melanin content will have disappeared. It is also known as vitiligo and Michael Jackson suffered from it, even though people said that he tried out skin whitening stunts.

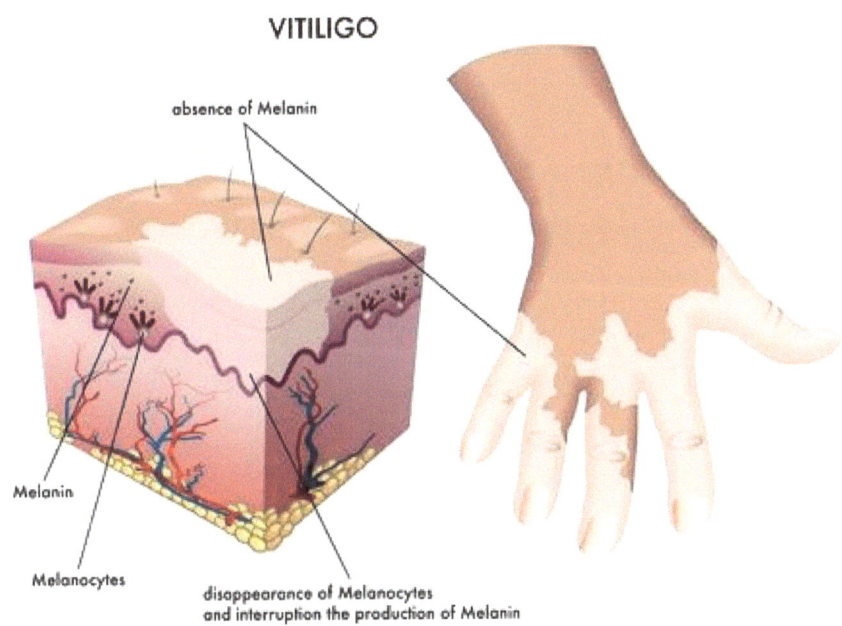

VITILIGO

absence of Melanin

Melanin

Melanocytes

disappearance of Melanocytes
and interruption the production of Melanin

For this, you are going to take a fistful of black gram and 10 g of an Herb mixture named Triphala powder- three fruit – it is made out of Terminalia chebula, emblica officianalis, and Terminalia bellirica.[1]

Put these into 125 g of water and allow to soak overnight. The next day, you are going to put the gram in a cotton cloth. The thrifala water was to give the gram more power. These are going to sprout in 24 hours. You are going to eat them slowly, chewing them well. This is a long-term cure, because you are going to get your system producing melanin again. It is going to take some months.

Along with this, you are going to eat bread made up of gram flour. Spread a spoonful of clarified butter on top of the hot bread before eating. Also, boost up your intake of gram in order to heal yourself faster.

Kidney Stones

People suffering from kidney stones should soak a fistful of gram dal lentils-gram without the outer cover – overnight in water. The next morning, you are going to eat this gram with honey, first thing in the morning. This is going to dissolve the kidney stones present in your kidney or in your bladder.

---

[1] https://en.wikipedia.org/wiki/Triphala

Corn – Zea Mays

What would one do without the bounty of corn?

No wonder in the ancient times, the Aztecs said that corn was brought to them by the gods, who taught them how to cultivate this gift of the gods. In ancient times, this plant was considered to be a symbol of plenty and prosperity, and even today, in many civilizations, it is a symbol of fruitfulness.

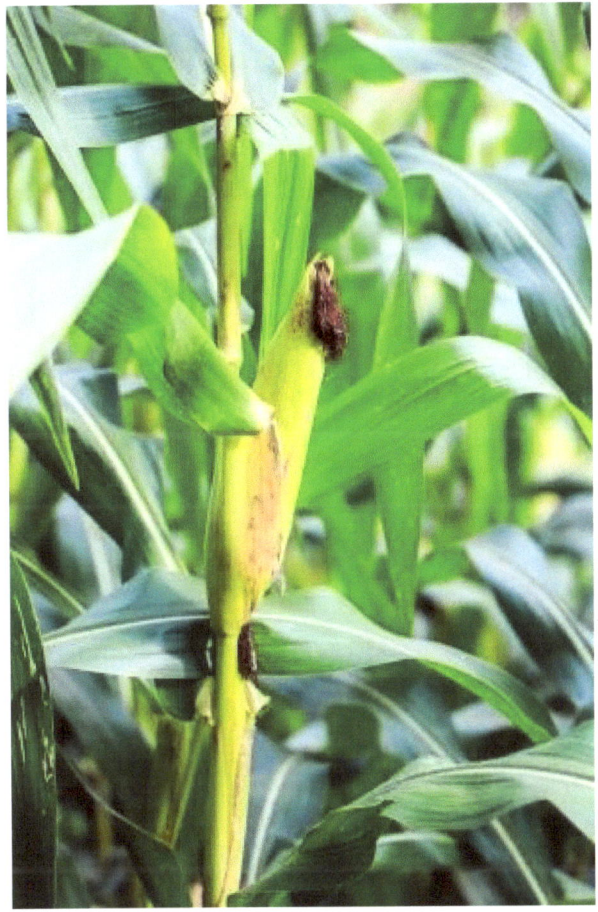

The corn seed is rich in vitamin B and proteins. The endosperm in the seed is rich in starch and the embryo has plenty of minerals, proteins and fat.

Traditionally, in the northern part of the Indian subcontinent, especially in the winter, corn flour is eaten with spinach/mustard and this is a traditional dish which every housewife/girl of the family needs to know how to cook, if she is to be considered a proper cook.

It is washed down with chunks of homemade butter and buttermilk. I remember once, as a child, being taken for horse riding by my father in our native town during the summer vacation and by the time, my younger brother and I had finished this enjoyable exercise and basic survival training, we came back home, as hungry as little wolves.

My grandmother had prepared cornbread with traditional green mustard, ground and cooked with spices, clarified butter, and onions. Hundreds of generations of youngsters before us must have come home after a hard days' work on the fields and fed this delicious tasty traditional dish.

I still remember the taste of that meal. No one has ever been able to duplicate it, especially the homemade butter and the buttermilk. My father told us to stop eating, when we grabbed the third piece of cornbread each, because he said we were still babies – I was seven and my brother, four – and would suffer from indigestion. But what a way to go!

According to researchers, in a research done in the 60s, this particular meal combination was one of the healthiest, in the world, because it had cereals, greens, and milk products, eaten every day, especially during the winter.

Corn on the cob is excellent for your digestive system. It also adds to the blood content. You may want to massage yourself with corn oil to have a healthy tissue growth.

How to Extract Corn Oil

If you do not have an oil extractor nearby in your city, you can take fresh on seeds, crush them a little, and put them in a glass container. Place them in the sun. The liquid quantity is going to evaporate in the sun, and you are going to see oil left behind in the container.

Put the soil in a glass bottle and use it for massage purposes. You can also mix a teaspoonful of this oil in any sherbet or squash you drink in order to get instant energy.

Whooping Cough

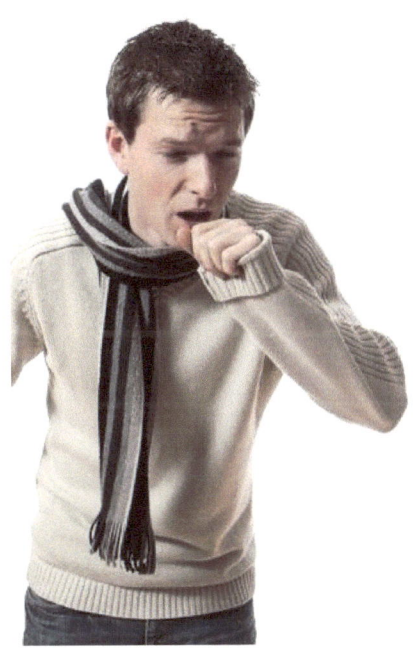

This is a remedy, told to me by my friend Joanna, whose grandmother told her many of these ancient remedies. You are going to take a corn cob and roast it until it is totally burned. Now you are going to grind this ash, and put it in a glass bottle. One fourth of a teaspoon full of this ash in one glass of hot water with a pinch of rock salt for taste has to be drunk four times a day, until you get rid of the whooping hacking cough.

Depression

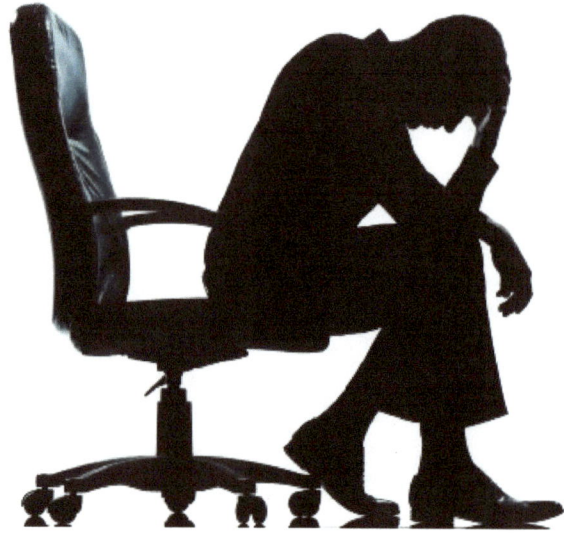

If you are suffering from stress, strain, tension, and depression, you just need to shell some corn cobs. You are now going to burn the corn cobs – without the seeds – and turn them into an ash.

Every day, you are going to take one fourth teaspoonful of this powder morning and night with one tablespoon full of honey. This is going to get rid of the depression, stress, tension, and loss of concentration problems.

Conclusion

This book has given you a knowledge of some time tested remedies, and how you can use them to keep healthy. There are plenty of traditional home remedies made up of cereals, found all over the world, but an extensive listing of all these remedies is going to take a lifetime of dedication.

This book is giving you just some time tested, and natural cures for some of these more common ailments. Remember that you need to eat unrefined grains and whole grains without the husk removed to keep healthy.

So take full advantage of nature's bounty, and live healthy, Live Long and Prosper!

Author Bio

Dueep Jyot Singh is a Management and IT Professional who managed to gather Postgraduate qualifications in Management and English and Degrees in Science, French and Education while pursuing different enjoyable career options like being an hospital administrator, IT,SEO and HRD Database Manager/ trainer, movie , radio and TV scriptwriter, theatre artiste and public speaker, lecturer in French, Marketing and Advertising, ex-Editor of Hearts On Fire (now known as Solstice) Books Missouri USA, advice columnist and cartoonist, publisher and Aviation School trainer, ex-moderator on Medico.in, banker, student councilor ,travelogue writer … among other things!

One fine morning, she decided that she had enough of killing herself by Degrees and went back to her first love -- writing. It's more enjoyable! She grams of already has 48 published academic and 14 fiction- in- different-genre books under her belt.

When she is not designing websites or making Graphic design illustrations for clients , she is browsing through old bookshops hunting for treasures, of which she has an enviable collection – including R.L. Stevenson, O.Henry, Dornford Yates, Maurice Walsh, De Maupassant, Victor Hugo, Sapper, C.N. Williamson, "Bartimeus" and the crown of her collection- Dickens "The Old Curiosity Shop," and "Martin Chuzzlewit" and so on… Just call her "Renaissance Woman" - collecting herbal remedies, acting like Universal Helping Hand/Agony Aunt, or escaping to her dear mountains for a bit of exploring, collecting herbs and plants, and trekking.

Check out some of the other JD-Biz Publishing books

Gardening Series on Amazon

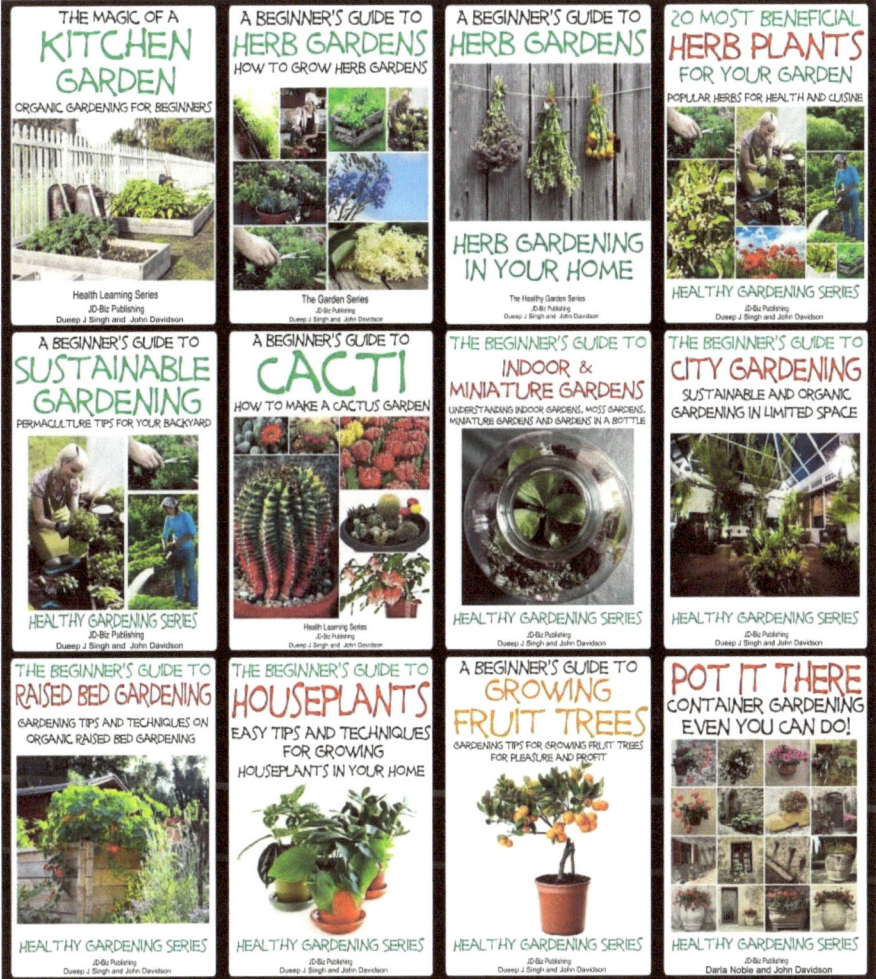

Download Free Books!

http://MendonCottageBooks.com

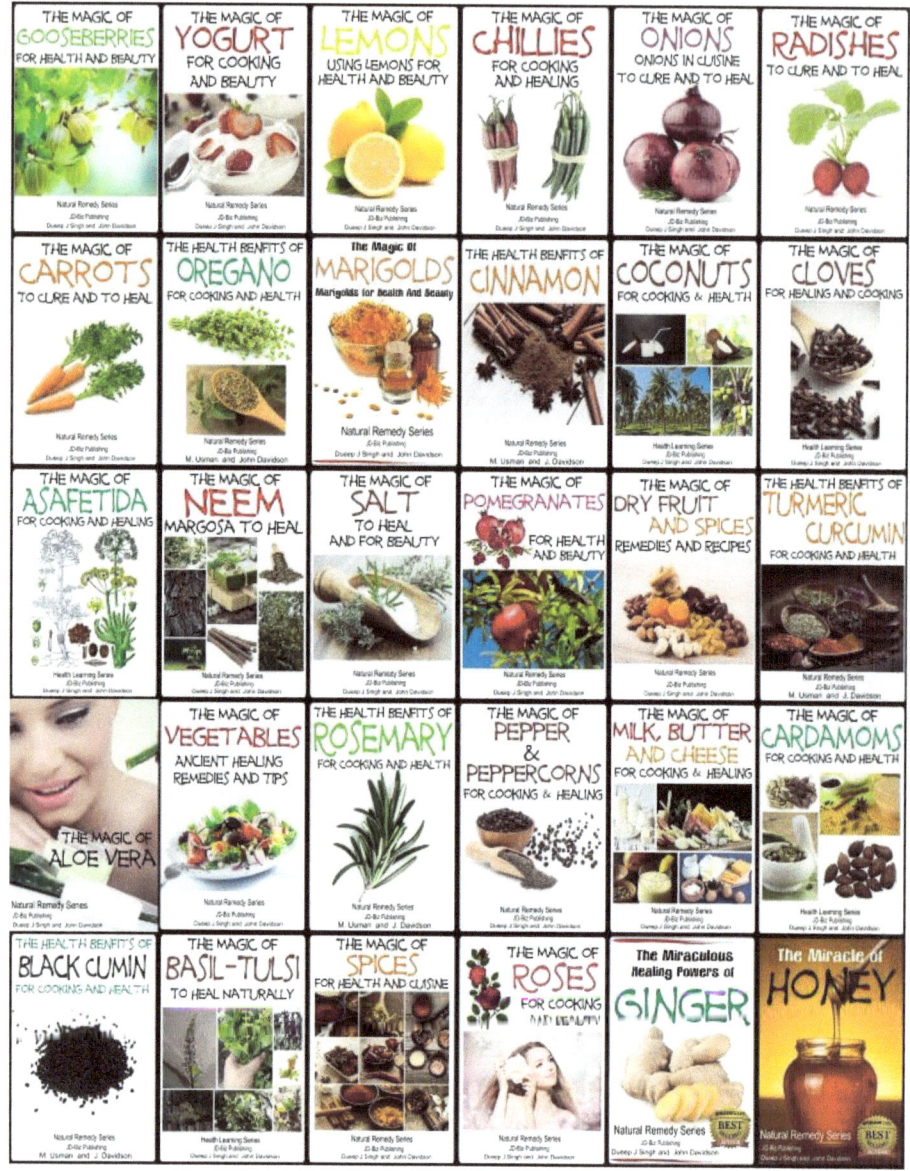

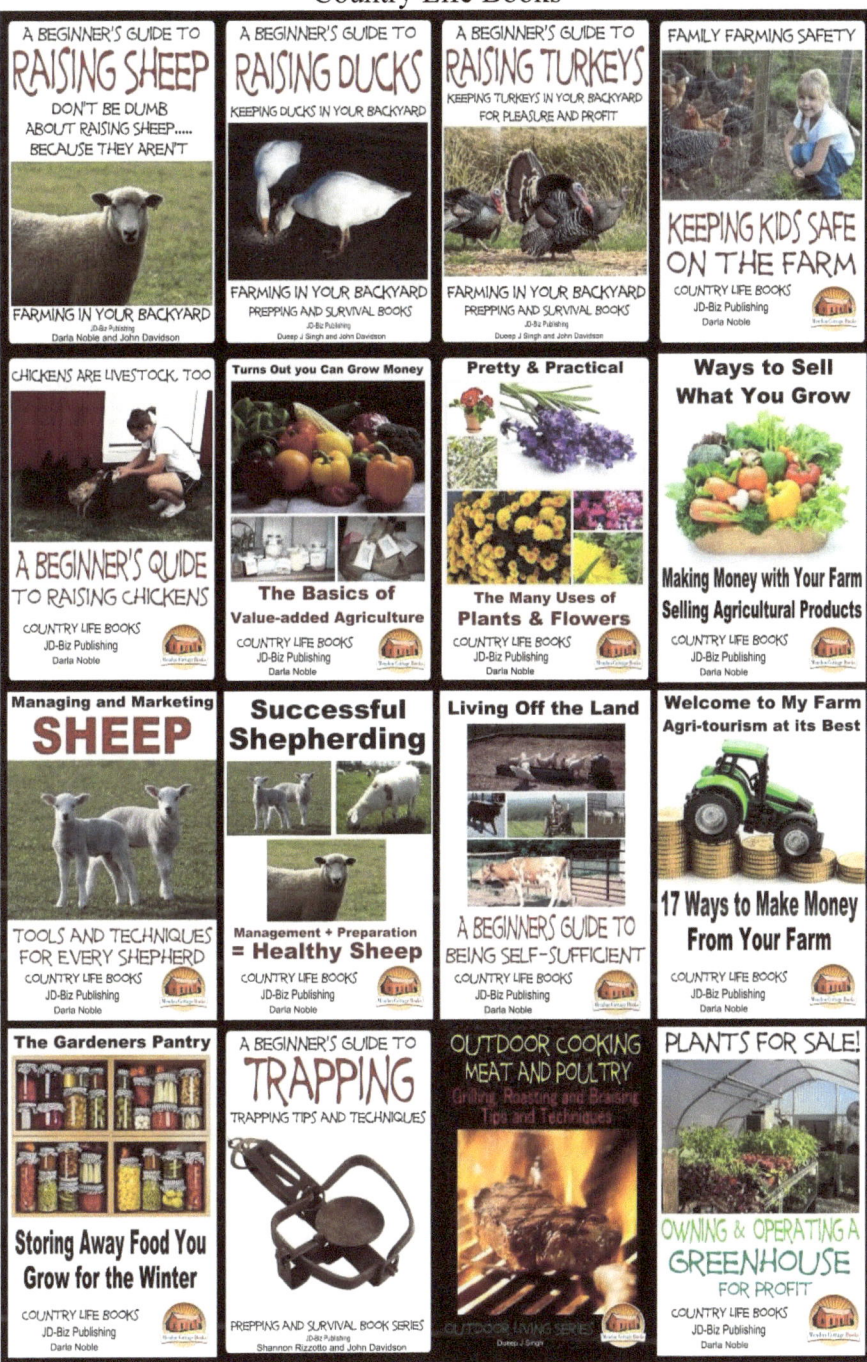

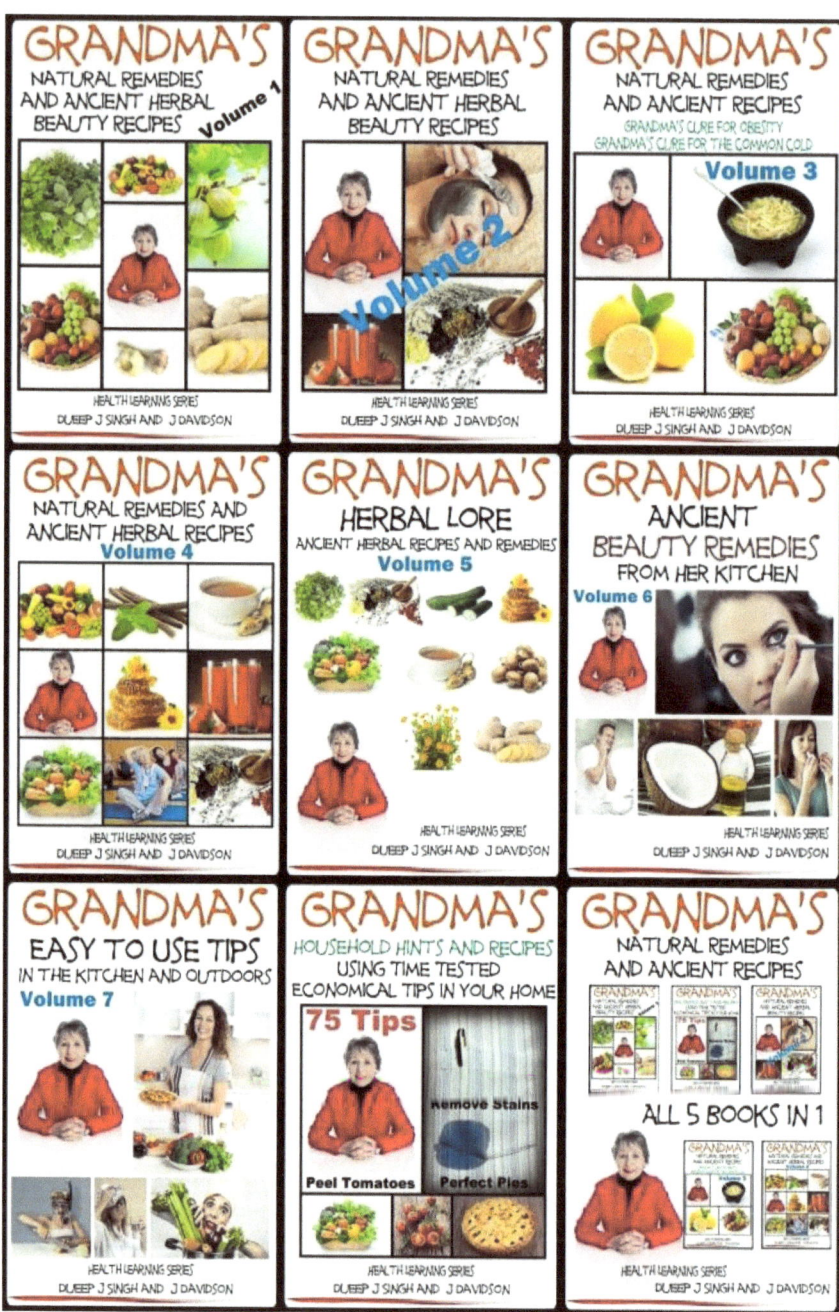

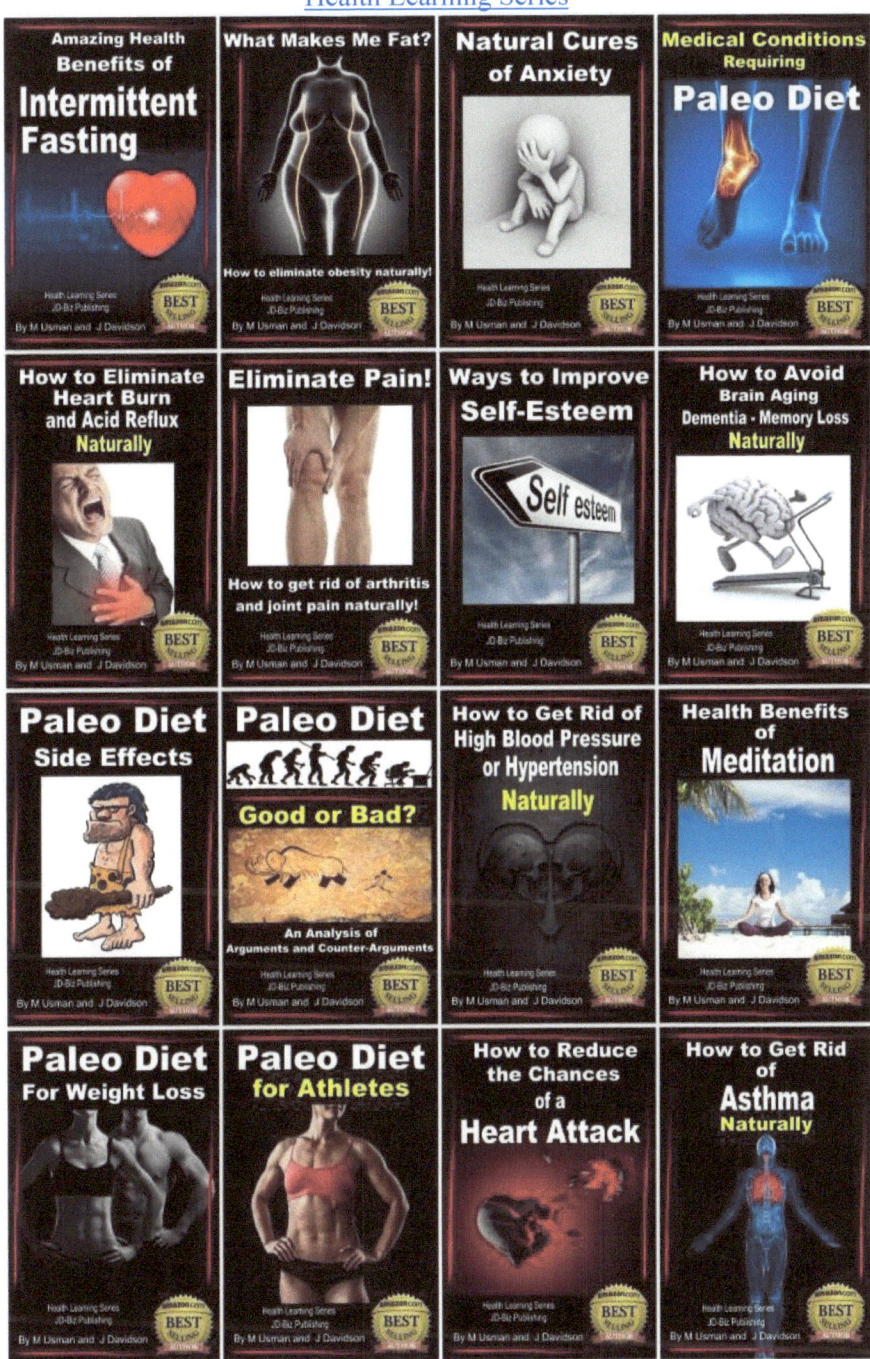

Amazing Animal Book Series

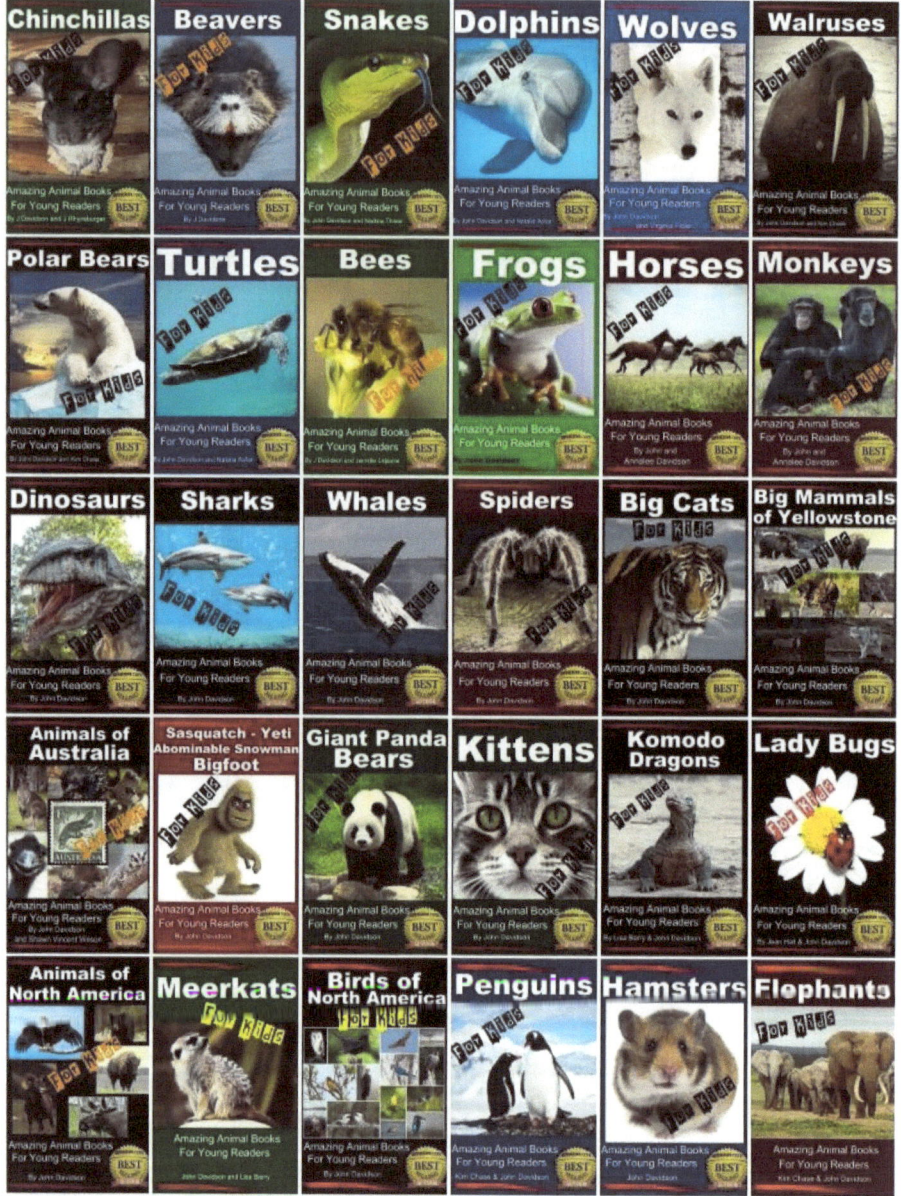

Learn To Draw Series

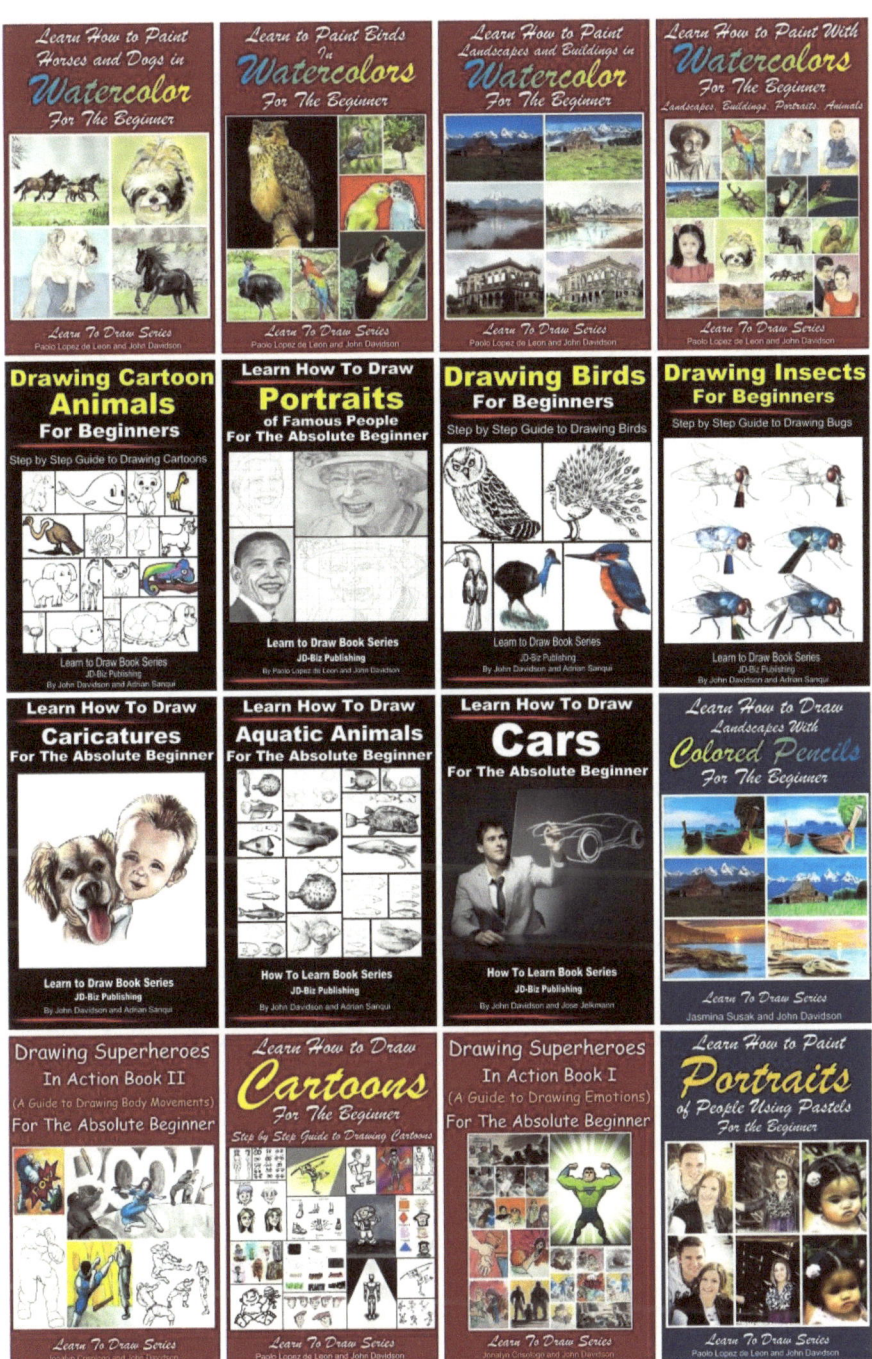

How to Build and Plan Books

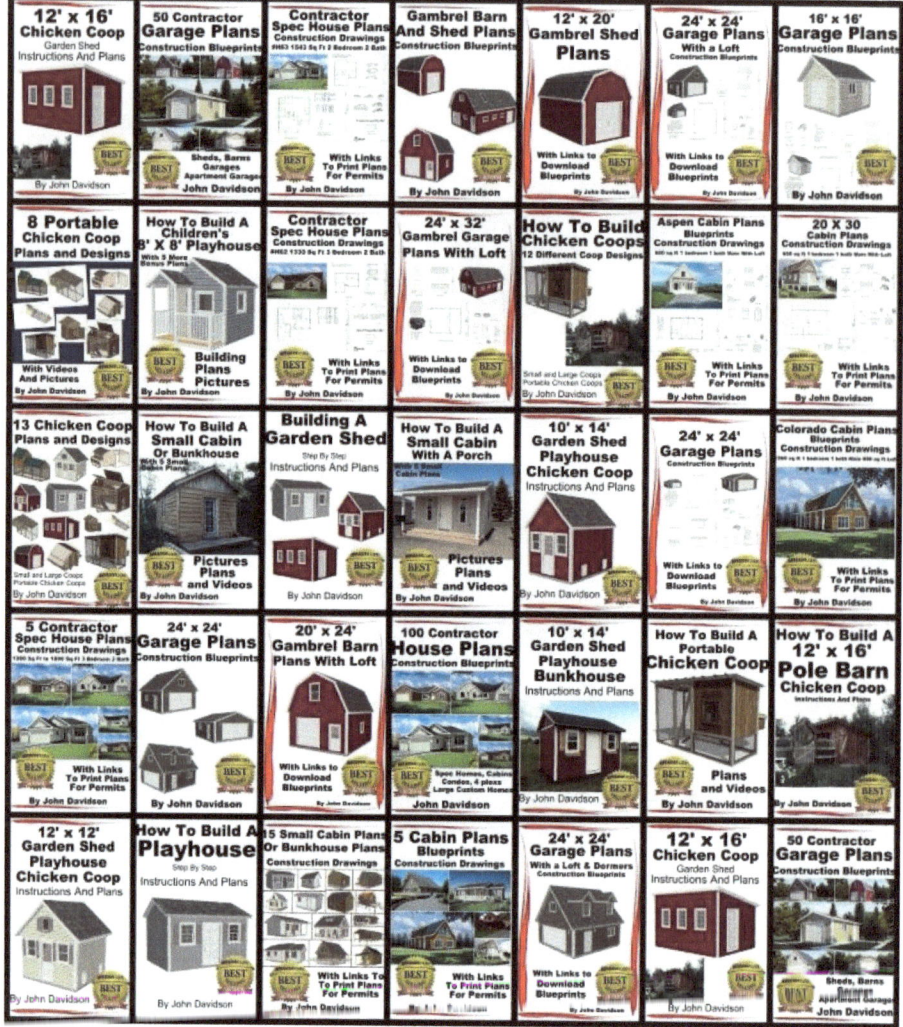

Entrepreneur Book Series

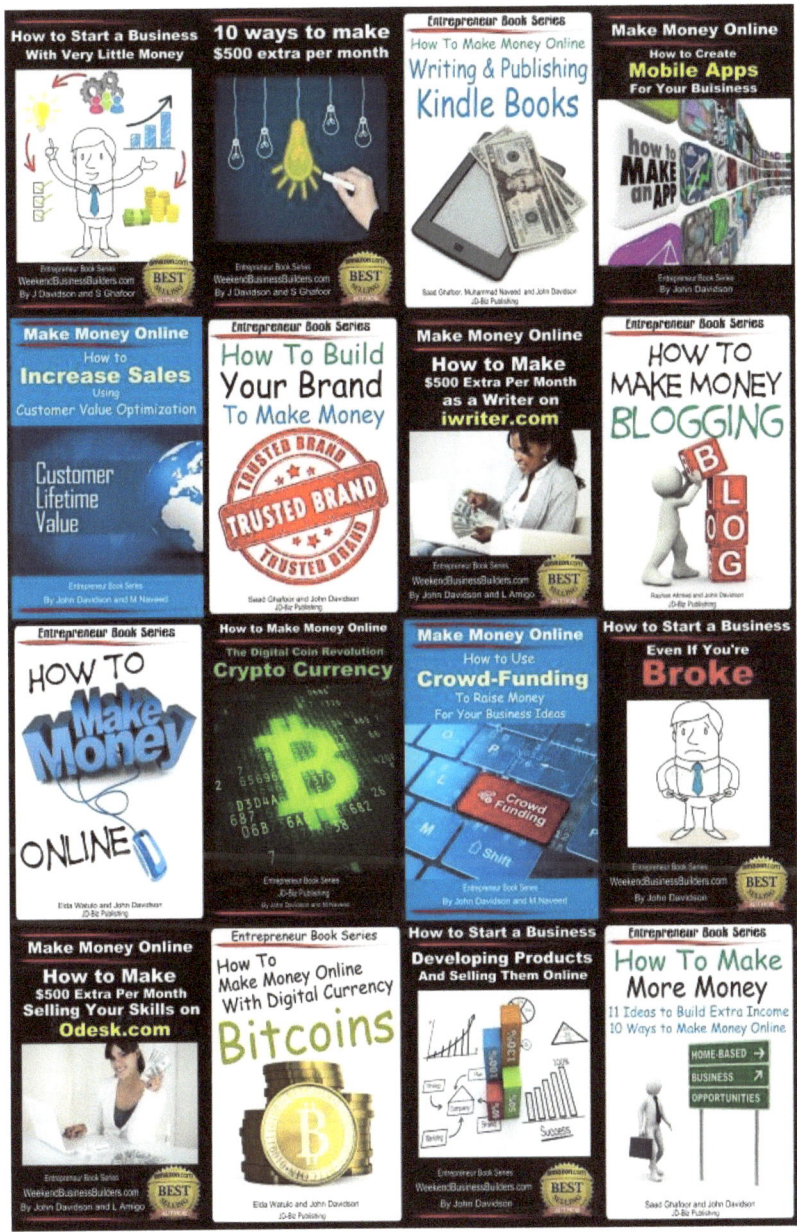

Our books are available at

1. Amazon.com

2. Barnes and Noble

3. Itunes

4. Kobo

5. Smashwords

6. Google Play Books

Download Free Books!

http://MendonCottageBooks.com

Publisher

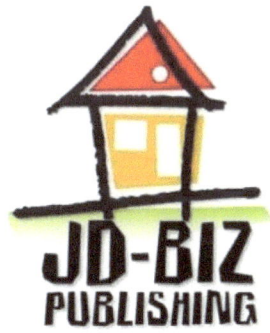

JD-Biz Corp

P O Box 374

Mendon, Utah 84325

http://www.jd-biz.com/

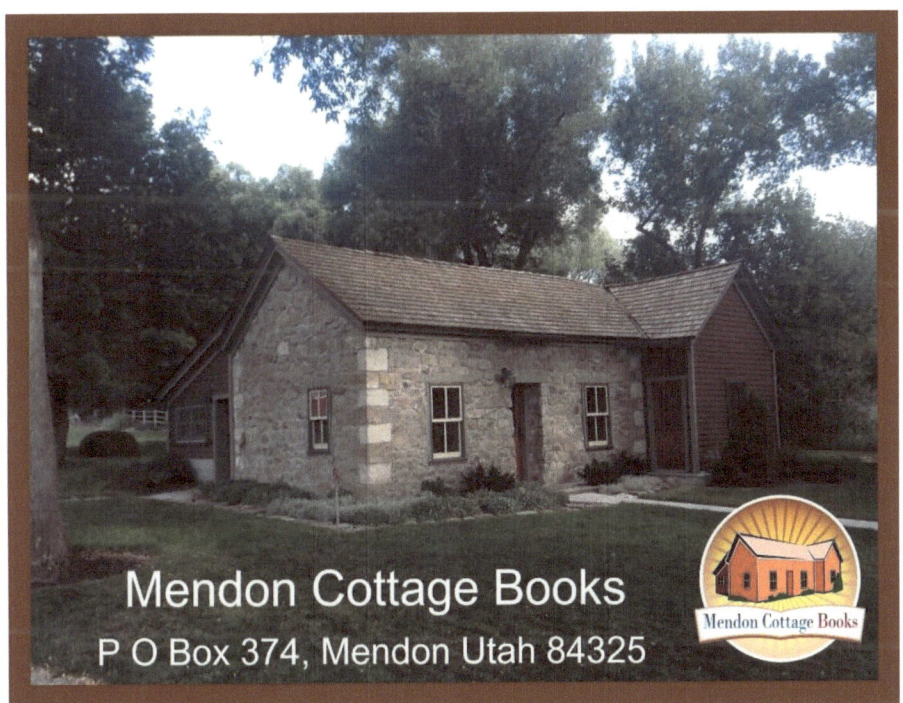

Mendon Cottage Books

P O Box 374, Mendon Utah 84325

www.ingramcontent.com/pod-product-compliance
Lightning Source LLC
Chambersburg PA
CBHW050822290526
45792CB00001B/228